7 DAY DETOX

EAT HEALTHY, EAT LIGHT, LOSE UP TO 7 POUNDS

D0229647

JACQUELINE WHITEHART

PEPIK BOOKS

Pepik Books

York

www.52recipes.co.uk

Text © Jacqueline Whitehart 2017

Jacqueline Whitehart asserts her moral right to be

identified as the author of this work.

A catalogue record for this book is

available from the British Library.

ISBN: 978-0-9955318-5-7

7 DAY DETOX

A NEW APPROACH

Welcome to Jacqueline's **7 Day Detox** Programme.

The menu is designed to give you 3 proper meals a day so you won't go hungry.

Nutritionally Balanced

Each day of the diet is nutritionally balanced so you are getting plenty of lean protein, good fats, smart carbs and a variety of fruit and vegetables. Latest science supports the addition of SIRT foods like green tea and dark chocolate into the diet. These really do curb your hunger pangs and make the diet easier to maintain.

Although calorie counting isn't at the forefront of the diet, the menu is planned so that you eat the least calories on the first 2 days and this is stepped up for the next 2 days and finally stepped up again for the remaining 3 days. The diet just gets easier and easier as you go along. This is to make sure you get great results and stick to the diet for the full week.

"Fantastic food, very easy to follow plan and above all, fun to cook with simple ingredients."

Neelam

Working Together

This diet is not about starving yourself, it's about sticking to a plan and working together to achieve the same goal.

I am committed to making sure **everyone** who joins the programme get the best from it. I provide help and support throughout.

"Jacqueline is supportive and encouraging every step of the way."

Ali

I don't know any other plan that gives a *"real, human helping hand"* from the comfort of your own home.

1   I will send you helpful emails every day (sign up here - www.52recipes.co.uk/7days/)

2   There's a very friendly Support Group on Facebook (join here - https://www.facebook.com/groups/jacquelines7daydetox/)

3   And I'm ALWAYS at the end of an email, for queries big and small (j@52recipes.co.uk)

PS. You can start anytime, no set start dates

INTRODUCTION

Over the last 5 years, I have become something of a diet expert. After experimenting (and failing) with many diets as I tried to lose weight after the birth of my third child, I started to approach dieting more scientifically and look at the whys and wherefores rather than just following whatever diet took my fancy that day. In 2012 I became one of the leading experts in the 5:2 diet, writing three best-selling guides to the diet.

I also discovered that my cookery knowledge could be used to create unique and healthy recipes that people really loved. In 2015 my love of 5:2 began to fade. Don't get me wrong, I still think it's a great diet if you can follow it, but the self-sacrifice on the diet days gets harder as time goes on and the results diminish greatly. In 2015 I was also asked by my publisher HarperCollins to look into the benefits of a new science-based food trend called SIRTfoods.

My approach has always been to research and self-experiment first and if it works for me to start writing recipes and simple guidelines that help other people too. I have found that these special superfoods really do curb your appetite and help you lose weight. I have used this knowledge to add plenty of SIRT foods into the programme.

The result of my years of research is this

specially designed programme, where you don't need to think about balancing the food groups and getting the best diet-friendly foods. I have tailored a programme that works and is easy to follow for just about everyone.

Don't just take my word for it. The *7 Day Detox* really does get great results:

"An impressive 8lb weight-loss. People have noticed I have lost weight, my clothes fit better and I feel great."
Sadie

"The diet plan has changed my way of cooking and eating habits. I love the way I feel. I have bucket loads of energy. Thank you Jacqueline, you have changed my life."
Kim

"I didn't believe it was possible to lose so much weight in one week. It's all been done eating healthy, clean food and the odd treat too."
Anna

The *"7 Day Detox"* programme is designed to be followed strictly for 7 days with impressive weight-loss results. I have drawn on the best elements of 5:2 dieting, although don't worry we will never be as extreme as 5:2 and there will always be 3 meals a day. Also included are the best and simplest SIRT foods. As before, I have tried and tested the different elements of the diet and double-checked all the recipes before beginning.

Yours,

Jacqueline

PREPARATION

It's as easy as 1-2-3 to prepare for the "7 Day Detox" plan.

A week before...

A week before you start you need to think about three things:

1 **buy one or two specialist ingredients (either online or from a health food shop)**

2 **cut back your caffeine intake**

3 **reduce your alcohol consumption**

You can get a *PREPARATION CHEAT SHEET* and *SHOPPING LIST* by joining the Email Support Group here - **www.52recipes.co.uk/7days/**

There are just 3 ingredients that you may not have come across before: chia seeds, malt extract and white tea. The first is chia seeds. These are tiny, virtually tasteless black seeds, similar to poppy seeds in appearance. We use chia in the granola recipe. Chia seeds are rich in protein and fibre and make a noticeable difference to your hunger levels after breakfast. They help the granola keep you full until lunchtime and beyond. These are now readily available in supermarkets.

The second ingredient is malt extract. If you are of a certain age, you may remember this as something you were fed by the spoonful as a small child. Malt extract is used in the granola. Malt extract is a natural maltose sweetener. It is less 'sweet' than sugar but doesn't give you the sweet highs and lows of normal sugar. As a bonus, it has a rich malty taste that adds flavour to your cooking.

Malt extract is hard to find in supermarkets at present, but can be found at health food shops. It can also be called Barley Malt Syrup. Rice Malt Syrup is very similar and can be used instead. If all else fails, substitute the malt extract for maple syrup in the granola recipe.

The final specialist ingredient is white tea. You may well be able to find this in the supermarket and is also available through health food shops. Although flavoured varieties might end up being your preference, I would start with a 'plain' good quality version.

Please get in touch as soon as you can if there are ingredients that are not easily accessible for you. Suitable alternatives can definitely be found but they will vary country by country. By letting me know what's difficult for you, I can help you source the right foods for you and will also help me assist others in the future.

The next thing to think about in the week before you start the "7 Day Detox" programme is to cut back your caffeine and alcohol intake. Reduce your caffeine so you don't get withdrawal symptoms during the diet, such as headaches and grumpiness.

"I thoroughly enjoyed the experience and broke some bad habits (coffee and alcohol) too. When I started to see my results there was no looking back."

Helen

During the 7 day programme, the only caffeine you will drink is white/green tea. Two cups of white tea are equivalent to 1 cup of coffee or 2 cups of tea. If you regularly drink more than this quantity of tea and coffee, try and gradually cut down to one or two cups a day. You may also want to give the white tea a try before you start the programme so you know what to expect.

"A great side effect was that I kicked a bad caffeine habit and drank more fluids."

Carolyn

The diet is alcohol-free for three reasons: alcoholic drinks contain empty calories that we don't need; when we drink will-power tends to go out of the window so we eat more and finally, we sleep less well when we've been drinking. If you sleep less then you are more tired the next day, and a common side-effect of tiredness is to comfort eat. By cutting back on alcohol in the week leading up to the diet we are improving our sleep patterns and getting ourselves feeling good and ready to diet.

"All addictions to processed food and alcohol have disappeared. The joy of simple food that is easy to cook. Adding herbs and spices gives flavour without piling on the pounds."

Caroline

A few days before...

A few days before you start you need to purchase the ingredients needed from the shopping list and start preparing some of the meals in advance so you are ready to go. All the breakfast and lunch recipes can be made in advance.

"Being part of the 7 Day Detox has been such an achievement. The recipes are simple and tasty. The shopping list is a godsend."

Sandra

You can get a 'PRINT OUT AND TAKE TO THE SHOPS' Shopping List here - **www.52recipes.co.uk/7days/**

GETTING STARTED

Think about when you want to start the diet. Pick a week with lots to keep you busy but little or no social events. This is a plain and simple week.

Many people find that the best day to start the programme is on a Monday, giving you time to gather ingredients and prepare meals over the weekend. You should choose whichever day works best for you and your schedule.

The day before you start you should record your starting weight. Then you can weigh-in optionally at the start of day 3 (Wednesday) and day 5 (Friday). The final weigh-in should be the morning of day 8 – just after the diet has finished.

Don't Diet by Yourself

Research shows that you are much more likely to succeed in your diet with support.

BUT I also understand that some people don't want to be a 'social dieter' and chat to others about their weight-loss ups and downs.

That's why the programme includes **TWO** incredible options to help you follow the *"7 Day Detox"* programme. These extras are totally **FREE**, and you can choose to do one or the other or both.

There's plenty of interacting and cheering each other on via the facebook group:

Facebook

Search 'Jacqueline detox' on Facebook and I'll add you right in.

If you don't fancy the social side, then I highly recommend the unique and free motivational email course that comes along with the plan. Get tailored emails every day during your '7 Day Detox'...you choose your start date.

Email

Sign up here: **www.52recipes.co.uk/7days/**

"No pressure, no chat, just a helping hand."

And of course, everyone who joins either the facebook group or email support plan will be able to message me personally and privately with any questions or concerns.

Can't decide? Do both.

THE SEVEN DIET STEPS

Every diet must have its rules and this one has seven guidelines to keep you on the straight and narrow.

1 Drink green or white tea every day

Try to drink at least 2 cups a day. Experiment with brands and flavours in the week before the diet as that will help you adjust.

2 Don't drink alcohol

For the seven days of the diet, you should cut out alcohol in your diet. Why? Think how even one small glass of wine might affect you. Firstly, is one glass ever enough? You relax and enjoy and suddenly your glass is empty. The temptation for a top-up is almost unavoidable. Secondly, any alcoholic drink will lower your resistance to extra foods and snacks. Remember it's only for 7 days!

3 No red meat

Red meat is higher in saturated fat than chicken or fish. What's more, the type of saturated fat found in red meat, especially processed red meat, has been proven to cause added stress to the body. Saturated fat found in dairy is better for you.

4   Fresh real ingredients

The "7 Day Detox" programme encourages healthy patterns that will help you keep the weight off with healthy 'real' recipes. Processed food is digested quicker and can leave you prone to unnecessary hunger.

5   No bread, pasta or wheat-based foods

Calories from bread and pasta are empty calories. They don't fill you up and you are soon hungry again. They are digested quicker than other carbohydrates and are more easily converted to fat cells. What's more, in many people, wheat can lead to bloating and digestive problems. Cut them out for the week of the programme and see if you notice the difference.

6   Low sugar

Sugar or sweetened foods are harder to resist than others. You are naturally drawn to sweeter foods. But if you cut back to very little sugar then your sweet cravings will be reduced. After eating sugar, you might notice a sugar-high: a surge of energy as the sugar is turned into energy. But a high is always followed by a low. Within 2 hours of eating sugar, your body will be calling out for more food and more sugar. Break this cycle and you'll lose weight much quicker.

7   Cut caffeine

Coffee and tea are great. I love my morning cuppa – it's the best drink of the day. But our dependence on these drinks gets in the way of our diet goals. So, for the 7 days of the diet, the only caffeine should come in the form of green or white tea. If you're a caffeine addict, you might suffer from a few withdrawals symptoms such as headaches and grumpiness. It is much easier to follow the programme if you cut down coffee and tea in the week before the diet. Take a look at 'Preparation' for more info on how to do this.

Why is white/green tea so vital?

Green and white teas are the only source of one of the most powerful sirtuin bio-actives, catechin. Catechins are so potent that only a small quantity, one small cup, triggers fat metabolism and reduces oxidative stress.

- Appetite suppressant
With a cup or two of white tea inside you, you will really notice the difference in terms of hunger pangs. You should find that you don't think about food between meals.

- A little bit of caffeine

A cup of white tea contains about half of the caffeine you'd find in a cup of coffee or similar caffeine you'd find in a cup of black tea. This caffeine is just enough to combine with the catechins to have an even more powerful fat-burning effect. This is the optimum way to convert fat to muscle.

- More energy

Hard to measure but definitely there, the catechins give you a little natural buzz that makes starting the day a smidgeon easier.

- Cumulative effect

The power of white tea keeps on giving and two cups of white tea is better than one cup, three cups are better than two cups, etc.

- Zero calorie

White tea is naturally calorie free. It doesn't need sugar or sweetener and gives you energy without the calories.

Learning to love white tea

A lot of people say that they dislike the taste of white tea. I agree it's not a taste that most people will instantly like – especially if you've never tried it before. But a bit of perseverance pays dividends here. The first cup may be horrible, the fourth just doable, the tenth nearly enjoyable and by the second week of regular drinking, it should be pleasant and refreshing. I am a total convert now.

If you find it truly difficult, start with two cups a day: one before or with breakfast and one mid-morning. Pour a small weak cup of tea and wait for it to cool to easy drinking temperature. Then just drink it quickly like medicine. Treat it like a necessary evil if required, and I promise you it will get easier.

If you prefer green tea, then this has the same amazing health benefits. In my experience it's just a bit too 'grassy' so I have settled on white tea. This is a little bit more expensive but has a cleaner taste. You will also notice a difference in brands. If you don't like one brand, try another as they are all subtly different. If you pay a bit more for a quality brand, then you should get a fresher taste. There are also several flavoured green teas that might turn out to be 'the one': mint, lemon and jasmine are all common and there are many wonderful sounding green fruit teas available too. For white tea, my preferred brands are clipper and teapigs.

The tea ritual for people that hate tea rituals

Boil the kettle and then leave for 30 seconds so that it goes 'off the boil'. Pour over the tea leaves or tea bag. Leave to brew for 1–4 minutes, depending on the brew strength required. Start off with a short brewing time (under a minute for me) and build up gradually. Loose leaf tea is really tasty but you need a special teapot, so if you're happy with teabags, stick to them. Also, a glass or delicate china cup complements the subtle flavour. Recycling your teabags (twice) or tea leaves (4 times) is positively encouraged. The second cup often tastes even nicer than the first. This is also a great way to make your tea go further and be cheaper per cup.

A TYPICAL DAY

Start the day with a simple glass of water. Before you do anything else, pour yourself a nice cold glass of water (medium-sized is fine) and drink it before you think of tea, food or anything else. Why? Because you will always be dehydrated after sleep and any early morning hunger could be just a lack of water. It will help balance your body and will start to wake up your system more effectively than a cup of coffee or tea.

Next on the list is a cup of green or white tea. I know some of you will find this hard. For years and years, I have always had a 'normal' cup of tea with milk to start the day and it is a bit of a shift. But, it's only for a week, it gets easier every day and, if you have prepared your body by reducing your tea and coffee intake in the week leading up to the diet, then you won't feel any caffeine withdrawal, just a light refreshing buzz from the small (but significant) amount of caffeine in the green tea.

Next…wait. Try to have your breakfast at least an hour after waking, but not more than 2½ hours. So, if you get up at 7 am, you should have breakfast between 8 am and 9.30am. This is the optimum time because if you eat it too early, you won't have fully woken up and will not be properly hungry. You are in danger of getting hungrier earlier too. Likewise, if you have breakfast too long after getting up you will be famished and the breakfast won't fill you up, leaving you with possible cravings and the tendency to overeat later.

After your deliciously filling granola, you should find that you are nicely full until lunchtime. But if you do feel yourself weakening, top up your white/green tea levels and that should give you a boost.

Lunch is a relatively light meal, so make the most of it and savour the warmth and flavours. Make sure you drink a glass or two of water as well and finish off with a cup of white tea.

Come mid-afternoon you might start to feel hungry and at this point, you need to just make sure your fluids are topped up, possibly have a few frozen grapes, and if you are on day 3 or beyond have a small portion of dark chocolate. Make sure you eat it slowly and allow it to dissolve in your mouth so you really enjoy it. Mid-afternoon can be a danger time when it's just too easy to reach for a biscuit. Stay strong and focus on what's important. Keep busy, stay away from the kitchen, and start to think about your delicious dinner which is only a short while away...

Dinner is a relatively early meal on this diet, aim to eat between 5 and 7 pm as this is when your body needs it the most. Again, if possible, savour this meal. Take your time to prepare and serve it – don't just wolf it down. If you have other people's food to prepare as well, then I suggest making their food first and eating yours in relative peace afterwards.

Finally, we reach the evening which, in truth, is the part of the day I struggle with the most. You've eaten all your food for the day, and the evening is distinctly lacking in excitement. It's often not a case of real hunger – more like boredom and habit. Many of us reach for whatever treats we can find in the evening and this is one of the most common causes of slow but steady weight gain. The most important thing we can do is break this habit over the 7 days of the diet. It will get us a long way towards achieving our weight-loss goal and enable us to maintain the weight-loss when the programme is over.

Tips for diet evenings

- Be strict with yourself and remind yourself what it is all for.
- Distraction, distraction, distraction. Keep away from the kitchen and wherever you hide your treats. Watch TV, read a book, go to bed early.
- Stay active. Go for a walk and get some fresh air.

- Seek support from the Facebook group. They'll make sure you step away from the wine glass!

Keeping yourself hydrated

You need to say 'No' to diet drinks or anything with artificial sweeteners. We are trying to stick to real foods without chemical enhancement so rule these out for now.

Water and more water

I know it's boring but water is refreshing and good for you.

Sparkling water with ice and lemon

Make a glass of water so much more of an event by serving chilled sparkling mineral water with ice and lemon. This also works with still mineral water and even tap water.

Fresh lime soda

This is another way to jazz up a simple glass of water naturally. Place several ice cubes in a long tall glass. Halve a fresh lime and cut off one generous slice. Squeeze the rest of the lime juice into the glass. Add your choice of still or sparkling water and top with the slice of lime. This is extremely refreshing and only adds 2 calories so knock yourself out!

Fruit teas and more

Apart from the white tea you drink during the day, you may find a fruit tea, or a chamomile, peppermint or similar is just the ticket when you want something un-caffeinated and warming. There are so many to choose from these days so stick to your favourite if you have one or try a selection if you're new to them.

Time for a treat...

Believe it or not, there are a few healthy treats that make their way into this diet. This is because if you remove everything sweet from your diet you'll start to feel withdrawal from the sweet stuff and you might just fall off the wagon. So here are your treats for the week – and yes for 5 out of the 7 days you can eat lovely, lovely chocolate.

Frozen grapes

Red/black grapes are a great source of SIRT superfoods which can help you with food cravings. There is fruit sugar in grapes so you can't have too much of them. This is where freezing grapes come in. You can set the portion size in advance and the frozen grapes take longer to eat and give a close approximation of sweets.

You can have a 10 grape portion of frozen red grapes as often as once a day from day one onwards. Place up to 10 grapes in a small container or freezer bag. Freeze. Take out a pack when you're ready to eat. It's that simple!

70% Dark chocolate

Dark chocolate contains lots of SIRT superfoods which curb your hunger and the small amount of sugar in the chocolate fulfils your sugary cravings. Don't be tempted to go for an 85% dark chocolate as this is too bitter to properly satisfy. Buy one 100g (4oz) bar of chocolate and this is your allowance for the week – no more no less. Keep days one and two chocolate free as these are your lightest days but know that treats are coming for the rest of the week.

Here's how I do it. Buy one 70% dark chocolate bar. My preferred choice is Green & Blacks as this divides neatly into 10 lines of 3 squares. On day 3, open the bar up and break or cut into 10 evenly sized pieces. Wrap each portion in cling film or foil and put away ready for when they're needed. I think one mid-afternoon and one in the evening is great as this is when we most need our sweet hit. There's enough for 2 portions a day for every day from day 3 to day 7. Or if you prefer you can save them up and have even more towards the end of the week. Just make sure you enjoy every mouthful extremely slowly. Take a small bit, pop it in your mouth and allow to melt on your tongue. You could even try the old fruit pastilles trick and don't chew.

A little bit of fruit

If you fancy a little bit of fruit mid-afternoon to stave off hunger pangs, then you can replace a chocolate portion with a choice of fruit on any day from day 3 onwards. Allowed fruits are apples, oranges, satsumas, strawberries (4), raspberries (10), blackberries (10), blueberries (25) and kiwi. On each day from day 3, you can have 2 portions of dark chocolate OR 1 portion of dark chocolate and 1 portion of fruit.

MEN: TAILORING THE 7 DAY DETOX

I don't want to lie to you. I have created this programme primarily for women. And over 95% of people who follow this programme will be women. But this plan can be as successful, if not more so, for men as women. In fact, men are even more likely to achieve 7 pounds or more weight-loss.

We do need to make a few changes to make the plan perfect for you. This is because men need more calories to maintain a stable weight. Cutting back on this programme will be harder as it may be too restrictive, leaving you prone to extreme hunger and exhaustion.

There is a simple fix that can be applied across the programme. We are just going to add some more protein. The rule of thumb is that to each meal we add 50% more protein. So, if a recipe suggests 100g chicken, you should use 150g. To make it even simpler to follow, all the protein in the recipes has been adjusted. For example, *100g (150g M) chicken breast, diced*, denotes that the recipe requires 100g chicken for women and 150g chicken for men.

If you are a man following the 7 Day Detox Programme, please let me know how you get on. I would love to hear from you.

EXERCISE

We don't want to forget about exercise during this week. But also it is not our top priority. 80% of weight-loss comes from diet alone and actually stressing our bodies too much with intense exercise will leave us hungry and more likely to binge eat. This weight-loss plan works so well because we are decreasing the stress on our bodies and waking up our metabolism. But I'm not suggesting even for a moment that we give up on existing exercise routines or ignore exercise during the week.

Exercise when done right and in moderation helps us to burn fat. Have a look at the three options and choose which best suits you at the present time. This means looking at yourself honestly and if you'd like to be a regular exerciser but are actually a sporadic or occasional exerciser then look at the occasional exercise routine. Maybe next time you check you'll be a regular exerciser. Type of exercise, the length of training and frequency of exercise are all key to a good balance.

During the week we will concentrate on 'sweaty' exercise, with the aim being to exercise 3-5 times during the last 5 days of the programme.

It is important to note that you should not do any exercise except very gentle exercise such as walking during the first two days of the plan. This is because these are the lightest days and exercise could make you weak.

In the 5 days, you should look to do 'sweaty' exercise between three and five times. Examples of sweaty exercise include running and walking, swimming, cycling, aerobic or dance-based exercise classes. Any exercise that includes weights or weighted machines is likely to be a strength exercise and should be avoided for the duration of the programme. If these are the classes you love, it's just a week and your strength and muscles will not suffer for the rest. In fact, you will be reinvigorated when you start again.

Why should you avoid strength exercises during the programme?

The reason is very simple. This is a fat and weight-loss programme. It's all about getting rid of excess fat. Strength exercises make you stronger and fitter and improve your muscle tone. It comes after weight-loss. If you do strength exercises during the plan, you will be increasing muscle instead of losing weight.

The banana quick-fix
For emergency use only! If within an hour of exercise you feel weak or you get severe hunger pangs then add in a small banana (or half a large banana). That should do the trick and keep you on track without upsetting your weight-loss goals. The banana quick-fix is allowed for all types of exerciser.

Days 1 and 2 of the plan (for all types of exerciser)

During the first 2 days of the programme, it is important not to over-exercise as these are the lightest days in terms of calories consumed. If you exercise hard on these days you may feel light-headed or find the plan difficult to maintain. So take a break and make sure the only exercise you do is a very gentle. Gentle exercise is relaxing and makes you feel great. The simplest of all is a half an hour walk. But a gentle swim or a yoga class would be perfect too.

Why is simple walking so beneficial?

Walking is a fantastic exercise for many reasons. Perhaps the most important is that it lowers your stress hormones. This not only makes you feel better but also encourages your body to burn fat, not sugar.

Your metabolic response to walking means that each time you walk (or swim or do yoga) you are reducing your insulin resistance by a tiny bit and enhancing your ability to burn fat. So never dismiss walking as 'not proper exercise', embrace and enjoy it.

If you are a regular exerciser...

You should consider yourself a regular exerciser if you do a higher intensity (sweaty) exercise 3 or more times during days 3-7 of the programme. The best time to exercise is the morning (the earlier the better) as this will burn fat more efficiently and you shouldn't increase your hunger pangs too much. The optimum length of time for exercising is 35-50 minutes.

If you are an occasional exerciser

You should consider yourself an occasional exerciser if on average you do some proper exercise about once a week. If that exercise is cardio, for example going for a run or an aerobics class, then continue with the class and consider adding in up to two other cardio exercise sessions per week.

Your aim is to do 1-3 sessions of cardio exercise during days 3-7. Your exercise routine should last between 30-45 minutes.

You should also consider adding some non-strenuous exercise into your routine. These are the same as suggested for days 1 and 2. Ideally, you should try to do non-strenuous exercise on any day during days 3-7 when you are not doing cardio exercise. If you don't believe this is helping you at all, rate your mood at 4 pm on a day when you exercise and a day when you don't and I bet you'll see an improvement on an exercise day.

If you do not exercise

Never fear, I am not going to ask you to force you into lots of exercise with which you are uncomfortable. As I said before 80% of weight-loss is down to diet so changing your routine for this plan is not necessary. What I would suggest is that you do 30 minutes of walking at least four times during the programme. It would be even better if you tried to do this every day. Think about how or where you could do this. Is it getting off the bus at an earlier stop? A walk round the town at lunchtime? A stroll with the dog (or someone else's) at the end of the day? However you do it, the walk should be no less than 30 minutes long and at a brisk pace. In simple terms, this means that you are exerting yourself but you can still carry on a conversation.

Suitable Cardio Exercise for all types of exerciser

Please don't consider this list to be absolutely everything. I live in York and we're always a little bit behind the times in terms of new classes etc. If your preferred exercise is not on the list but is not weight-bearing and could be considered 'sweaty' then you're good to go.

- Cycling
- Running
- Swimming
- Spinning

- Rowing
- All aerobics including aqua aerobics
- Zumba, Sh'bam, FitSteps or any dance-based class
- Body combat
- Grit cardio
- Circuit training
- Cardio-based HIIT

SHOPPING LIST

Meat and Fish	Chilled and Frozen
4 chicken drumsticks 3 chicken breasts 250g (9oz) raw king prawns (king shrimp) 1 salmon fillet	Butter 2 large pots natural yogurt 1 large egg 60g/2oz smoked salmon Soya (soy/edamame) beans (fresh or frozen)

Fruit and Vegetables	Store Cupboard
1 white onion 1 red onion Large piece fresh ginger 3 shallots 1 head garlic 4 carrots (1 large, 3 small) 1 small parsnip Celery Butternut squash (½ or 300g/11oz prepared) 1 head broccoli (200g/7oz) 1 cucumber 3 medium tomatoes 2 green (bell) peppers 1 red (bell) pepper 1 green chilli 1 red chilli Spring onions (Scallions) Shiitake mushrooms Small pack beansprouts Baby leaf spinach Pak Choi New potatoes Mange tout (Snow peas) 2 limes 2 lemons Red grapes	Olive oil Extra virgin olive oil Mild olive oil Cornflour (Cornstarch) Light Soy sauce English mustard Tomato puree (paste) Peanut butter Red wine Mayonnaise Rice wine or mirin Whole peppercorns 3 x can chopped tomatoes 1 x can kidney beans 1 x can butterbeans 200g/7oz cooked Basmati rice White or green tea Brown sugar Cocoa powder Jumbo oats Flaked almonds Chia seeds Malt extract/Barley Malt Syrup* (not Coeliac) Maple syrup (Coeliac only) Dark chocolate chips 1 100g/4oz 70% dark chocolate

Herbs and Spices			
Fresh	**Dried**	**Spices**	
Parsley Coriander/ Cilantro Fresh mint	Bay leaves Thyme Dried mixed herbs	Chilli powder Ground cumin Paprika Smoked paprika	Gr Turmeric Gr Cinnamon Cloves (whole) Gr Ginger

SHOPPING LIST (V)

Chilled and Frozen	
4 medium eggs	Black olives
1 large egg	Butter
Feta cheese	2 large pots natural yogurt
Paneer cheese	Soya (soy/edamame) beans
Tofu	(fresh or frozen)

Fruit and Vegetables	Store Cupboard
1 white onion	Olive oil
1 red onion	Extra virgin olive oil
Large piece fresh ginger	Mild olive oil
3 shallots	Cornflour (Cornstarch)
1 head garlic	Light Soy sauce
4 carrots (1 large, 3 small)	English mustard
1 small parsnip	Tomato puree (paste)
Celery	Mayonnaise
Butternut squash (½ or	Rice wine or mirin
300g/11oz prepared)	Whole peppercorns
1 cucumber	
2 green peppers	3 x can chopped tomatoes
2 red peppers	1 x can kidney beans
1 green chilli	1 x can blackbeans
1 red chilli	1 x can chickpeas
1 courgette (zucchini)	100g/3½oz cooked Basmati rice
Spring onions (Scallions)	White or green tea
Shiitake mushrooms	Brown sugar
Small pack beansprouts	Cocoa powder
2 bags Baby leaf spinach	Jumbo oats
Pak Choi	Flaked almonds
New potatoes	Chia seeds
Mange tout (Snow peas)	Malt extract/Barley Malt
	syrup* (not Coeliac)
2 limes	Maple syrup (Coeliac only)
2 lemons	Dark chocolate chips
Red grapes	1 100g/4oz 70% dark chocolate

Herbs and Spices			
Fresh	**Dried**	**Spices**	Gr Turmeric
Parsley	Bay leaves	Chilli powder	Gr Cinnamon
Coriander/	Thyme	Ground cumin	Gr coriander
Cilantro	Dried mixed	Paprika	
Fresh mint	herbs	Smoked paprika	

Note that although almost all of the ingredients are readily available in supermarkets or local stores, malt extract is a little harder to find. I purchased malt extract from Holland & Barrett in the UK. It can also be called Barley Malt Syrup.

If you can't find malt extract, rice malt syrup is a good alternative. If you can't find either of these (or if you are coeliac) try using maple syrup instead.

7 DAY MENU AT A GLANCE

	Monday	Tuesday	Wednesday	Thursday	Friday	Saturday	Sunday
	Chia Choc Granola with natural yogurt	Chia Choc Granola with natural yogurt	Chia Choc Granola with natural yogurt	Chia Choc Granola with natural yogurt	Chia Choc Granola with natural yogurt	Chia Choc Granola with natural yogurt	Chia Choc Granola with natural yogurt
	Chicken & Root Vegetable Broth OR Root Vegetable Broth with Tofu	Chicken & Root Vegetable Broth OR Root Vegetable Broth with Tofu	Vegetable Chilli	Mexican Chicken Soup OR Mexican Bean Soup	Vegetable Chilli	Mexican Chicken Soup OR Mexican Bean Soup	Vegetable Chilli
	Smoked Salmon & Soft-boiled Egg on Spinach & Cucumber Salad OR Feta Salad with Olives & Soft-boiled Egg	Chinese-style Chicken with Pak Choi OR Mushroom & Blackbean Stir-fry	Chicken Cassoulet OR Moroccan Spiced Eggs	Lightly Spiced Prawns (Shrimp) with Vegetable Rice OR Fresh Saag Paneer	Peanut Butter & Lime Prawns (Shrimp) OR Feta Stuffed Red Peppers	Chicken Cassoulet OR Moroccan Spiced Eggs	Creamy Baked Salmon with New Potatoes & Mange Tout OR Bean Burgers with New Potatoes & Mange Tout

RECIPES

This is a 3 meal a day diet so over the seven days that's 21 meals. The key to making the diet workable is making sure the meals are as simple to prepare as possible. Breakfast, for example, is a delicious granola that you make a batch of at the start of the week. Lunches are split over 2 to 3 days and dinners are quick to prepare and last one or two nights.

"Not feeling hungry was the best. The recipes were simple and tasty and didn't need loads of specialist ingredients."

Jo

There are 4 big recipes for this diet. The first is *Chia Choc granola*. A delicious and incredibly filling breakfast with which you will start every day of the diet.

"I will be using the recipes forever."

Joanne

Lunch for the first two days is an amazing *Chicken and Root Vegetable Broth*, which is a cleansing soup to make you feel invigorated and encourage fat breakdown.

"I haven't really felt hungry and think the recipes are so good! Will be using them again."

Sally

The other two lunches - *Vegetable Chilli* and *Mexican Chicken Soup* - are both designed to really stave off those hunger pangs. These core recipes are designed to give you excellent nutrition and to be as filling as possible while low in calories. Every day from the start you will have a 'proper' and varied dinner.

The breakfast and lunch recipes are all designed to be made in advance and kept in an air-tight container (granola) or the fridge/freezer so that you don't need to do lots of cooking during the week. In fact, all these recipes are so quick and easy to cook you may find they'll become a staple of your everyday cooking. Note that any ingredient with a revised quantity denoted by 'M' is the quantity for Men only. Women following the plan should use the quantity not in brackets.

Speedy Recipe 'Little Helpers'

If you're not used to cooking from scratch for every meal, you may find the level of preparation daunting. There's a couple of really easy fixes that can help you no end ... without cheating and without reducing the quality of the food you are cooking. Want to know the answer? It's frozen pre-chopped vegetables! Don't scoff! If you want to cut your prep time in half and save on wastage then these will really help.

- **Frozen Chopped Onions**
  A lot of recipes start with 'an onion, peeled and chopped'. So if you can use these instead you not only save time, but stop the onion tears as well. A smaller portion

is perfectly good to replace shallot too so that's practically every meal sorted. Use a generous handful (2 heaped tablespoons) to replace on onion or a much smaller handful (1 tablespoon) to replace a shallot.

- **Frozen (Bell) Peppers**

Peppers are used in several recipes in the plan so these can be a godsend. You tend to get mixed frozen peppers rather than individual colours. There's a simple rule to follow with mixed peppers. Green peppers taste different from the other colours and should be separated. So if a recipe says green peppers pick out the green ones. But if a recipe says red pepper use red, yellow or orange but avoid the green ones. Watch out if you're planning on having the *Feta Stuffed Peppers (V)* as these require a whole red pepper rather than chopped.

- **Garlic Puree (paste)**

You can get different types of chopped or frozen garlic but I honestly find garlic puree in a tube to be the best. It can be used as a substitute in all the recipes in the programme and is a fantastic time saver. I really like Gia Garlic Puree and I just squeeze a bit in (roughly 1 teaspoon) every time a clove of garlic is asked for.

- **Frozen Butternut Squash**

For the *Vegetable Chilli*, frozen butternut

squash is revolutionary. Butternut squash is one of the most annoying vegetables to chop and prepare with its rock hard skin and messy seeds. In fact, you can replace all the vegetables in the chilli with frozen options and it becomes ridiculously quick and easy to prepare.

CHIA CHOC GRANOLA

221 calories • 303 cals with yogurt

This amazing recipe is an absolute diet staple. Clever use of ingredients means that this recipe is more protein and fibre-rich than other cereals. And it contains only complex carbs and sugars. As a result, when combined with 100g/4oz (150g/5oz M) natural yogurt this makes a really tasty and satisfying breakfast. Energy is released slowly and it is guaranteed to keep you full and curb hunger pangs for at least 4 hours. One batch makes 7x45g(1³⁄₄oz) portions.

Note: Malt Extract can be replaced with barley/ rice malt syrup or maple syrup

MAKES 7 PORTIONS • READY IN 30 MINS

200g (7oz) jumbo oats
....
20g (¾oz) flaked almonds
....
20g (¾oz) chia seeds
....
2 tbsp (30ml) mild olive oil
....
10g (1/3oz) butter
....
1 heaped tbsp (40g/1½oz) malt extract
....
40g (1½oz) dark chocolate chips
....

- Pre-heat the oven to 160C/140C fan/325F. Line a large lipped baking tray with greaseproof (waxed) paper or a silicone sheet.
- In a large mixing bowl, combine the oats, almonds and chia seeds.

- Place the olive oil, butter and malt extract in a small non-stick saucepan. Heat very gently, stirring until the butter has melted and the ingredients have combined. Do not allow to bubble or boil.

- Remove from the heat and pour into the oats. Mix together until all the oats have a light coating of the sweet butter. When fully coated, tip out onto the prepared baking tray and distribute over the tray. Allow some gaps and a few clumps to form on the tray rather than an even spread. Bake in the pre-heated oven for 18-20 minutes.

- Remove from the oven and allow to cool completely on the tray. When cool, lightly break up larger pieces of granola. Sprinkle the chocolate chips over. Transfer to a lidded jar or air-tight container and store until needed.

CHICKEN AND ROOT VEGETABLE BROTH

93 calories

This light and refreshing broth still provides a good source of protein in the chicken.

MAKES 2 PORTIONS • READY IN 2 HOURS

1 onion, peeled and roughly chopped

1 carrot, peeled and chopped

1 stick celery, trimmed and chopped

2 (3 M) chicken drumsticks, skin on

1 litre (4 cups) water

8 whole peppercorns

1 tsp salt

1 bay leaf

1 small parsnip, peeled
and finely chopped

1 small carrot, peeled
and finely chopped

1 clove garlic, peeled and crushed

1 tbsp light soy sauce

2 tsp English mustard

2 spring onions (scallions),
trimmed and finely chopped

Pinch of freshly ground black pepper

- Take a large lidded pan and place the onion, carrot and celery inside. Add the peppercorns, salt and bay leaf.

- Pour in approximately 1 litre (4 cups) water and bring to a simmer. Place the lid on the pan and cook gently either on the hob or in a medium oven (170C fan/375F) for 1½ hours. Add the chicken drumsticks for the last 30 minutes of cooking time.

- Strain the broth through a sieve. Discard the vegetables and place the chicken drumsticks on a plate. Leave to cool for 15 minutes or until the drumsticks can be handled comfortably.

- Return the broth to the pan. Add the parsnip, carrot and garlic to the broth and simmer for about 15 minutes until tender.

- Remove the skin from the drumsticks and pull the chicken off the bone. The chicken will just fall off the bone after its long cooking time. Discard the bones, skin and waste and separate the good chicken into 2 portions.

- Add the soy sauce, English mustard and spring onions (scallions) to the broth and stir. Add the pepper and taste to check the seasoning. Divide the broth between 2 containers equally. Refrigerate the broth and the chicken separately until needed.

- When you are ready to eat the broth, reheat a portion until lightly bubbling. Then add the chicken and warm through.

ROOT VEGETABLE BROTH WITH TOFU (V)

107 calories

The vegetable broth is packed full of flavour and the tofu adds extra protein.

MAKES 2 PORTIONS • READY IN 2 HOURS

1 onion, peeled and roughly chopped

1 carrot, peeled and chopped

1 stick celery, trimmed and chopped

1 litre (4 cups) water

8 whole peppercorns

1 tsp salt

1 bay leaf

1 small parsnip, peeled
and finely chopped

1 small carrot, peeled
and finely chopped

1 clove garlic, peeled and crushed

1 tbsp light soy sauce

2 tsp English mustard

2 spring onions (scallions),
trimmed and finely chopped

Pinch of freshly ground black pepper

100g (3½oz) (150g/5oz M) firm
tofu, cut into small chunks

• Take a large lidded pan and place the onion, carrot and celery inside. Add the peppercorns, salt and bay leaf.

- Pour in approximately 1 litre (4 cups) water and bring to a simmer. Place the lid on the pan and cook gently either on the hob or in a medium oven (170C fan/375F) for 1½ hours.

- Strain the broth through a sieve and discard the vegetables.

- Return the broth to the pan. Add the parsnip, carrot and garlic to the broth and simmer for about 15 minutes until tender.

- Add the soy sauce, English mustard and spring onions (scallions) to the broth and stir. Add the pepper and taste to check the seasoning. Divide the broth between 2 containers equally. Refrigerate the broth until needed.

- When you are ready to eat the broth, reheat a portion until lightly bubbling. Then add the tofu (50g/2oz per portion) and warm through.

MEXICAN CHICKEN SOUP

125 calories

This delicately spiced soup is warming and filling. Feel free to add a fresh chilli if you like it hot!

MAKES 2 PORTIONS • READY IN 1 HOUR

2 (3 M) chicken drumsticks

1 shallot, peeled and roughly chopped

I small carrot, peeled and roughly chopped

1 stick celery, trimmed and finely chopped

500ml (generous 2 cups) water

1x400g can chopped tomatoes

1 green (bell) pepper, deseeded and chopped

1 clove garlic, peeled and crushed

1 tsp dried mixed herbs

½ tsp paprika

½ tsp smoked paprika

¼ tsp turmeric

¼ tsp ground cumin

1 tsp salt

Freshly ground black pepper

1 tsp mild chilli powder

20g (¾oz) (handful) flat-leaf parsley, stalks removed and chopped

- Place the chicken drumsticks, shallots, carrot and celery in a large saucepan. Pour over the water and bring up to a simmer. Cook for 20 minutes, then remove the chicken drumsticks with a slotted spoon and set aside to cool.
- Add the chopped tomatoes, green (bell) pepper and garlic and bring back up to simmering point. Add the dried herbs, paprika, smoked paprika, turmeric, cumin, salt, black pepper and chilli powder, then simmer gently for 30 minutes.
- Remove the skin from the drumsticks and pull as much chicken as possible off the bone. Shred the chicken meat and return it to the pan. Remove from the heat and stir in the parsley.

MEXICAN BEAN SOUP (V)

123 calories

This delicately spiced soup is warming and filling. Feel free to add a fresh chilli if you like it hot!

MAKES 2 PORTIONS • READY IN 50 MINUTES

1 tsp olive oil

1 shallot, peeled and chopped

1 small carrot, peeled and roughly chopped

1 stick celery, trimmed and finely chopped

500ml (generous 2 cups) water

1x400g (14oz) can chopped tomatoes

1 green (bell) pepper, deseeded and chopped

1 clove garlic, peeled and crushed

1 tsp dried mixed herbs

½ tsp paprika

½ tsp smoked paprika

¼ tsp turmeric

¼ tsp ground cumin

1 tsp salt

Freshly ground black pepper

1 tsp mild chilli powder

½ x 400g (14oz) (full M) can blackbeans

20g (¾oz) (handful) flat-leaf parsley,

stalks removed and chopped
....

- Heat the oil in a large saucepan. Add the shallot, carrot and celery and fry gently for about 5 minutes.

- Add the water, chopped tomatoes, green (bell) pepper and garlic and bring a gentle simmer. Add the dried herbs, paprika, smoked paprika, turmeric, cumin, salt, black pepper and chilli powder, then cook gently for 30 minutes. Add the black beans, soaking liquor and all, and cook for a further 15 minutes.

- Stir through the parsley just before serving.

VEGETABLE CHILLI

198 calories

This is a classic filling recipe that really sets you up for the whole day. The kidney beans add a little bit of protein and some good carbs so get stuck in and enjoy. This can be made in advance and chilled/frozen in individual portions so can be ready to eat in minutes.

MAKES 3 PORTIONS • READY IN 45 MINUTES

300g (11oz) chopped butternut squash (this is the cut weight)

....

½ tsp ground cinnamon

....

2 tsp olive oil

....

1 red onion, peeled and chopped

....

1 green (bell) pepper, seeded and chopped

....

1 green chilli, seeded, sliced into rings

....

1 clove garlic, peeled and finely chopped

....

Zest and juice 1 lime

....

1 tsp mild chilli powder

....

1 tsp ground cumin

....

½ tsp paprika

....

½ tsp cocoa powder

....

1 tsp salt

....

1x 400g (14oz) can chopped tomatoes

....

1x400g (14oz) (2 M) kidney beans in water

....

Freshly ground pepper

....

- Preheat the oven to 220C/200C fan/425F.
- Place the butternut squash on a baking tray, sprinkle over the cinnamon and season generously with salt and pepper. Drizzle over 1 tsp of olive oil and toss through with your hands. Bake in the oven for 15–20 minutes, until just tender.
- Meanwhile, heat the remaining teaspoon of olive oil in a large pan and add the onion, green (bell) pepper and chilli. Fry gently for 5 minutes. Add the garlic and lime zest and cook for a further minute or two. Add the chilli powder, cumin, paprika, cocoa powder and salt. Stir through before adding the chopped tomatoes and kidney beans (including the water).
- Bring up to a gentle simmer and cook, lid off, for about 30 minutes. Add the butternut squash and lime juice and stir through gently. Taste and add salt and pepper to taste. Cook for a further 5 minutes. Allow to cool completely (this allows the flavours to develop) before storing as three individual portions. Reheat on the hob or in the microwave before serving.

SMOKED SALMON & SOFT-BOILED EGG ON SPINACH AND CUCUMBER SALAD

320 calories

This dish is simple to throw together and is stack full or protein to fill you up. Smoked salmon gives it a luxurious feel.

MAKES 1 PORTION • READY IN 10 MINUTES

1 large egg

2 tsp extra virgin olive oil

½ tsp English mustard

pinch of sugar

1 tsp mayonnaise

juice of half lemon

salt and pepper

40g (1½oz) baby leaf spinach

5cm (2in) cucumber, halved lengthways and sliced

60g/2oz (100g/3½oz M) smoked salmon, cut into small thin slices

- Heat a small pan of water to boiling. Using a slotted spoon, slowly lower the egg into the boiling water. Heat for 8-10 minutes depending on how well-cooked you like your egg. Remove from the water using the slotted spoon and cool in a bowl of cold water for a minute or two to stop the cooking process.

- Meanwhile, make the dressing by combining the olive oil, mustard, sugar, mayonnaise, lemon juice and salt and pepper in a small bowl.
- Arrange the spinach and cucumber over a plate and pour over half the dressing. Add the salmon. Peel the just cooled egg and quarter. Arrange the egg pieces over the salmon. Drizzle the rest of the dressing over. Serve immediately.

FETA SALAD WITH OLIVES AND SOFT-BOILED EGG (V)

334 calories

MAKES 1 PORTION • READY IN 10 MINUTES

1 large egg

2 tsp extra virgin olive oil

½ tsp English mustard

pinch of sugar

1 tsp mayonnaise

juice of half lemon

salt and pepper

40g (1½oz) baby leaf spinach

5cm (2in) cucumber, halved lengthways and sliced

40g/1½oz (60g/2oz M) feta cheese, cut into small cubes or lightly crumbled

4 black olives, halved

- Heat a small pan of water to boiling. Using a slotted spoon, slowly lower the egg into the boiling water. Heat for 8-10 minutes depending on how well-cooked you like your egg. Remove from the water using the slotted spoon and cool in a bowl of cold water for a minute or two to stop the cooking process.

- Meanwhile, make the dressing by combining the olive oil, mustard, sugar, mayonnaise, lemon juice and salt and pepper in a small bowl.

- Arrange the spinach and cucumber over a plate and pour over half the dressing. Add the feta and olives. Peel the just cooled egg and quarter. Arrange the egg pieces over the salad. Drizzle the rest of the dressing over. Serve immediately.

CHINESE-STYLE CHICKEN WITH PAK CHOI

354 calories

This delicious and filling stir-fry is perfect for the end of day two. You need a treat and this is perfect. It's really satisfying and will fill your kitchen with amazing smells.

SERVES 1 • READY IN 20 MINUTES

1 small skinless chicken breast (125g/4oz) (175g/6oz M), cut into strips

....

1 tsp cornflour (cornstarch)

....

1 tsp water

....

1 tsp rice wine

....

1 tsp tomato puree (paste)

....

½ tsp brown sugar

....

1 tbsp light soy sauce

....

½ clove garlic, peeled and grated

....

½ thumb (1cm/½in) fresh ginger, peeled and grated

....

1 tsp olive oil

....

½ tsp walnut oil

....

50g (1¾oz) shiitake mushrooms, sliced

....

2 spring onions (scallions), trimmed and shredded

....

100g (3½oz) pak choi, cut into thin slices

....

30g (1oz) beansprouts

....

- Toss the chicken pieces in the cornflour (cornstarch) until they are fully coated. Set aside. In a small bowl, stir together the water, rice wine, tomato puree (paste), brown sugar and soy sauce. Add the garlic and ginger and stir together.

- In a wok or large frying pan (skillet), heat the olive and walnut oils together on a medium heat. Add the chicken and stir-fry for 4-5 minutes each side until cooked through. Remove the chicken from the pan with a slotted spoon and set aside.

- Turn the heat up to high, add the shiitake mushrooms to the pan and stir-fry for 2-3 minutes until cooked and glossy. Then add the spring onions (scallions), pak choi and beansprouts and stir-fry until the pak choi has wilted.

- Reduce the heat to low, then stir in the cooked chicken. Add the sauce and allow the sauce to bubble around the chicken for a minute. Remove from the heat and serve immediately.

MUSHROOM AND BLACKBEAN STIR-FRY (V)

323 calories

This delicious and filling stir-fry is perfect for the end of day two. You need a treat and this is perfect. It's really satisfying and will fill your kitchen with amazing smells.

SERVES 1 • READY IN 20 MINUTES

1 tsp water

1 tsp rice wine

1 tsp tomato puree (paste)

½ tsp brown sugar

1 tbsp light soy sauce

½ clove garlic, peeled and grated

½ thumb (1cm/½in) fresh
ginger, peeled and grated

1 tsp olive oil

½ tsp walnut oil

50g (1¾oz) shiitake mushrooms, sliced

100g (3½oz) chestnut mushrooms,
washed and sliced

2 spring onions (scallions),
trimmed and shredded

100g (3½oz) pak choi,
cut into thin slices

30g (1oz) beansprouts

½ x 400g (14oz) (full M) can
blackbeans, rinsed and drained

- In a small bowl, mix the water, rice wine, tomato puree (paste), brown sugar and soy sauce. Add the garlic and ginger and stir together.

- In a wok or large frying pan (skillet), heat the olive and walnut oils together on a high heat. Add both types of mushrooms to the pan and stir-fry for 2-3 minutes until cooked and glossy. Then add the spring onions (scallions), pak choi and beansprouts and stir-fry until the pak choi has wilted.

- Reduce the heat to low, then stir in the blackbeans and add the sauce. Allow the sauce to bubble for a minute then remove from the heat and serve immediately.

CHICKEN CASSOULET

407 calories

This is a great 'all-in-one' dish. As you are eating this on two nights, Wednesday and Saturday, you should halve the cassoulet before adding the chicken and freeze or refrigerate the second half.

MAKES 2 PORTIONS • READY IN 1 HOUR

1 tsp olive oil

1 shallot, peeled, halved
and thinly sliced

1 small carrot, peeled and sliced

1 celery stick, trimmed and chopped

1 clove garlic, peeled and crushed

½ x 400g (14oz) can
chopped tomatoes

50ml (scant ¼ cup) red wine

200ml (generous ¾ cup) water

1 tsp dried thyme

1 heaped tsp brown sugar

½ tsp mild chilli powder

½ tsp smoked paprika

salt to taste

1 bay leaf

180g (6oz) new potatoes, 3-4
potatoes depending on size,
quartered lengthways

½ x 400g (14oz) can butterbeans
in water, drained

2 tsp (10g 1/3oz) butter

....

1 large or 2 small skinless chicken
breasts (approx. 200g/7oz total,
300g/11oz M), cut into cubes

....

200g (7oz) broccoli, steamed or
boiled (100g (3½oz) per meal/person)

....

- Add the shallots, carrot and celery to the pan, stir, replace the lid and cook gently for 5-8 mins until soft. Add the garlic, chopped tomatoes, red wine, water, thyme, brown sugar, chilli powder, smoked paprika, salt and bay leaf. Stir through, then add the new potatoes. Bring to a simmer and cook with the lid ajar for about 30 minutes.

- Add the butterbeans and divide the cassoulet into two portions. One for eating immediately and one to keep for the second night.

When you are ready to serve the cassoulet:

- Warm through the cassoulet until just bubbling.

- Heat half the butter in a frying pan (skillet). When the butter has melted, add half the chicken and fry for approx. 2 mins each side until golden brown but not cooked through. Add the chicken to the cassoulet. Bring to simmering point again and cook for 6-8 minutes or until the chicken is just cooked and tender. Remove the bay leaf before serving.

- Serve with broccoli on the side.

MOROCCAN SPICED EGGS (V)

394 calories

This unusual dish makes a lovely filling dinner.
Make the tomato sauce first and reheat it when
you are ready to cook the eggs. This dish is
served twice - Wednesday and Saturday night.

MAKES 2 PORTIONS • READY IN 50 MINUTES

1 tsp olive oil

1 shallot, peeled and finely chopped

1 red (bell) pepper, deseeded
and finely chopped

1 garlic clove, peeled and
finely chopped

1 courgette (zucchini), peeled
and finely chopped

1 tbsp tomato puree (paste)

½ tsp mild chilli powder

¼ tsp ground cinnamon

¼ tsp ground cumin

½ tsp salt

1 × 400g (14oz) can chopped tomatoes

1 x 400g (14oz) can chickpeas in water

small handful of flat-leaf parsley
(10g (1/3oz)), chopped

4 (6 M) medium eggs at
room temperature

- Heat the oil in a saucepan, add the shallot and
red (bell) pepper and fry gently for 5 minutes.

Then add the garlic and courgette (zucchini) and cook for another minute or two. Add the tomato puree (paste), spices and salt and stir through.

- Add the chopped tomatoes and chickpeas (soaking liquor and all) and increase the heat to medium. With the lid off the pan, simmer the sauce for 30 minutes – make sure it is gently bubbling throughout and allow it to reduce in volume by about one-third.
- Remove from the heat and stir in the chopped parsley. Divide the sauce into two portions.
- Preheat the oven to 200C/180C fan/350F.
- When you are ready to cook the eggs, bring one portion of the tomato sauce up to a gentle simmer and transfer to a small oven-proof dish.
- Crack two eggs on the side of the dish and lower them gently into the stew. Cover with foil and bake in the oven for 10-15 minutes. Serve the concoction in an individual bowl with the eggs floating on the top.

LIGHTLY SPICED PRAWNS WITH VEGETABLE RICE

383 calories

Although this has quite a few ingredients, the majority should be cupboard staples. If you don't like prawns/shrimp feel free to substitute with chicken (which you should add with the shallot rather than at the end).

Note also that you can use a packet of pre-cooked rice for this dish to make it even easier. I use Tilda brown basmati steamed rice.

MAKES 1 PORTION • READY IN 20 MINUTES

1 tsp olive oil

1 clove

1 bay leaf

1 shallot, chopped

½ red (bell) pepper, deseeded and chopped

1 clove garlic, peeled and thinly sliced

1 red or green chilli, deseeded and sliced (optional)

½ tsp mild chilli powder

½ tsp paprika

¼ tsp ground turmeric

¼ tsp ground cumin

¼ tsp cinnamon

½ tsp salt

1 fresh tomato, roughly chopped

30g (1oz) (50g/1¾oz M) frozen soya/edamame beans
1 tbsp water
125g/4oz (150g/5oz M) raw king prawns (king shrimp) (if frozen, cook for a little longer/defrost as per pack instructions)
100g (3½oz) cooked and cooled basmati rice
20g (¾oz) young leaf spinach, stalks removed
Small handful fresh coriander (cilantro), chopped (optional)

- In a wide lidded frying pan (skillet), heat the oil over a medium heat. Add the cloves and bay leaf. Add the onion and red pepper. Stir, turn the heat to low and place the lid on the pan. Cook for 5 minutes.

- Remove the lid from the pan. Add the garlic, chilli, chilli powder, paprika, turmeric, ground cumin, cinnamon and salt and fry for a further minute. Add the chopped tomatoes, soya beans and water. Replace the lid on the pan and cook gently for 7 minutes.

- Take the lid off the pan and remove the cloves and bay leaf. Add the prawns (shrimp) and cook until just pink. Then add the rice, stir thoroughly and warm through. Finally, stir through the spinach and coriander (cilantro) just before serving.

FRESH SAAG PANEER (V)

403 calories

Using fresh spinach gives a whole new to this curry-house favourite. You can use pre-cooked rice for this dish, such as Tilda steamed rice, to make it easier.

MAKES 1 PORTION • READY IN 20 MINUTES

1 tsp olive oil

....

100g (3½oz) (150g/5oz M)
paneer, cut into cubes

....

Salt and freshly ground black pepper

....

1 shallot, chopped

....

1 small thumb (2cm/1in) fresh ginger,
peeled and cut into matchsticks

....

1 clove garlic, peeled and thinly sliced

....

1 green chilli, deseeded
and finely sliced

....

50g (1¾oz) cherry tomatoes, halved

....

¼ tsp ground coriander

....

¼ tsp ground cumin

....

¼ tsp ground turmeric

....

½ tsp salt

....

50g (1¾oz) fresh spinach leaves

....

Small handful fresh coriander
(cilantro), chopped (optional)

....

100g (3½oz) cooked and
cooled basmati rice

....

- Heat the oil in a wide lidded frying pan (skillet) over a high heat. Season the paneer generously with salt and pepper and toss into the pan. Fry for a few minutes until golden, stirring often. Remove from the pan with a slotted spoon and set aside.

- Reduce the heat and add the shallot. Fry for 5 minutes before adding the ginger, garlic and chilli. Cook for another couple of minutes before adding the cherry tomatoes. Put the lid on the pan and cook for a further 5 minutes.

- Add the spices and salt, then stir. Return the paneer to the pan and stir until coated. Add the spinach and coriander (cilantro) to the pan together with the cooked rice and put the lid on. Allow the spinach to wilt for 1–2 minutes, then stir together thoroughly. Serve immediately.

PEANUT BUTTER AND LIME PRAWNS

362 calories

You make this amazing marinade for the prawns (shrimp) and then use it as a dipping sauce. Trust me – it's amazing!

SERVES 1 • READY IN 20 MINUTES

For the marinade:

Juice of ½ lime

1 tsp (10g (1/3oz)) peanut butter

1 tbsp water

½ tsp tomato puree (paste)

½ clove garlic, crushed

¼ tsp ground ginger

125g/4oz (200g/7oz M) raw king prawns (king shrimp)

For the rice:

100g (3½oz) cooked and cooled basmati rice

2 tomatoes, chopped

5cm (2in) cucumber, cut into small cubes

1 spring onion (scallion), finely chopped

Juice of ½ lime

Salt and pepper

• Combine all the marinade ingredients in a wide

bowl and stir together thoroughly. Add the king prawns (shrimp) and leave to marinate for 15-20 minutes.

- Place the cooked rice in a bowl and mash gently with a fork to remove any lumps. Add the tomatoes, cucumber and spring onion. Squeeze over the lime juice and season with salt and pepper. Stir well and leave for the flavours to develop.

- Remove the prawns (shrimp) from the marinade and shake off into the bowl so you don't lose any precious marinade. Place on kitchen paper to dry. Heat a frying pan (skillet) on a medium heat and add the marinade. Heat gently and allow to bubble for 2 minutes, adding a little more water if necessary, before transferring to a small bowl for dipping.

- Turn the heat up to high and add the prawns (shrimp). Fry for 3-4 minutes, stirring regularly until cooked through.

- To serve, place the rice on a plate and arrange the prawns (shrimp) over the top. Serve with the dipping sauce on the side.

FETA STUFFED RED PEPPERS (V)

380 calories

SERVES 1 • READY IN 20 MINUTES

1 red (bell) pepper, top removed,
halved and deseeded

1 tsp olive oil

½ x 400g (14oz) can cannellini beans

½ clove garlic, crushed

Juice of half a lemon

Salt and pepper

1 spring onion, finely chopped

4 cherry tomatoes, roughly chopped

Small handful fresh parsley, stalks
removed and finely chopped

40g/1½oz (60g/2oz M) feta cheese

4 black olives, sliced

40g (1½oz) baby spinach,
stalks removed

5cm (2in) cucumber, halved
and cut into semi-circles

- Preheat the oven to 240C/220C fan/450F.

- Rub the red (bell) pepper halves all over with the olive oil. Place face down on a small baking tray and bake in the oven for 10 minutes.

- Meanwhile, place the cannellini bean, garlic and lemon juice in a small bowl. Mash the beans roughly with the back of a fork and stir until well-combined. Season with salt and pepper. Stir in the spring onion, cherry tomatoes and parsley.

- Remove the peppers from the oven and turn them the right way up. Distribute the bean salad evenly between the two peppers. Crumble the feta over the top and add the olives. Return to the oven for a further 10 minutes.

- Serve the stuffed peppers straight from the oven on a bed of spinach leaves and cucumber.

CREAMY BAKED SALMON WITH NEW POTATOES AND MANGE TOUT

502 calories

A lovely way to end the week. This is a perfectly balanced and filling dinner.

MAKES 1 PORTION • READY IN 25 MINUTES

1 skinless salmon fillet, about 130g/4½oz (200g/7oz M)
....
salt and freshly ground black pepper
....
1 tsp olive oil
....
180g/6oz (about 4 medium) new potatoes
....
1 tsp mayonnaise
....
1 tbsp natural yogurt
....
1 tbsp rice wine
....
2 fresh mint leaves, finely chopped
....
2 spring onions (scallions), trimmed and sliced
....
100g (3½oz) mange tout (snow peas), trimmed
....

- Preheat the oven to 200C/180C fan/400F.

- Place the salmon fillet on a baking tray. Season with salt and pepper and rub the olive oil over the top. Bake in the oven for 16-18 minutes until just cooked through.

- Quarter the potatoes and steam or boil until tender.

- In a small bowl, combine the mayonnaise, yogurt, rice wine, mint leaves and spring onions (scallions). Leave for 5-10 minutes for the flavours to develop.
- Boil or steam the mange tout (snow peas) according to the pack instructions.
- Arrange the warm potatoes and mange tout (snow peas) over a plate. Lightly flake the salmon with a fork and arrange over the potatoes. Finally, pour over the dressing. Serve immediately.

BEAN BURGERS WITH NEW POTATOES & MANGE TOUT (SNOW PEAS) (V)

404 calories

Delicious and really quick to prepare.

MAKES 1 PORTION • READY IN 20 MINUTES

180g/6oz (about 4 medium)
new potatoes

½ × 400g (14oz) (full M) tin cannellini
beans, rinsed and drained

1 tsp tomato puree (paste)

1 tsp cornflour (cornstarch)

1 spring onion (scallion),
trimmed and chopped

½ clove garlic, peeled and crushed

½ tsp mild chilli powder

¼ tsp ground turmeric

Salt and freshly ground black pepper

1 tsp mayonnaise

1 tbsp natural yogurt

1 tsp rice wine

2 fresh mint leaves, finely chopped

2 spring onions (scallions),
trimmed and sliced

100g (3½oz) mange tout
(snow peas), trimmed

1 tsp olive oil

- Quarter the potatoes and steam or boil until tender. Add the mange tout (snow peas) for the last 4-5 minutes of cooking time. Drain and cover.

- Place the beans in a large bowl and use a potato masher or fork to thoroughly mash the beans. Add the tomato purée (paste), cornflour (cornstarch), spring onion (scallion), garlic, chilli powder and turmeric. Season generously with salt and pepper. Mix well.

- Divide the mixture into two portions and form into balls, then flatten a little to form a burger. If you have time, chill for 20 minutes or keep refrigerated until needed. The burgers will hold their shape slightly better if chilled but will be just as delicious if cooked straight away.

- In a small bowl, combine the mayonnaise, yogurt, rice wine, mint leaves and spring onions (scallions). Leave for 5-10 minutes for the flavours to develop.

- Heat the oil in a frying pan (skillet) over a medium heat. Add the burgers to the pan and cook for 3–4 minutes on one side. Turn with a fish slice and flatten a little more if necessary. Cook for a further 3–4 minutes until golden brown.

- Arrange the warm potatoes and mange tout (snow peas) over a plate. Place the burgers on the top. Finally, pour over the dressing. Serve immediately.

7 DAY PLANNER

Day One

Day one is the lightest day because you can still use stored energy from the day before. It's also the day when you'll feel the most motivated and possibly the day you will lose the most weight. Danger times when you might feel hungry and tempted are mid-afternoon and late evening. Get day one out of the way and each day gets easier from now on.

Chia Choc Granola

--

Chicken and Root Vegetable Broth
(Root Vegetable Broth with Tofu (V))

--

Smoked Salmon & Soft-boiled Egg on Spinach and Cucumber Salad
(Feta Salad with Olives and Soft-boiled Egg (V))

Day Two

Day two is also relatively light but the Chinese Chicken Stir-fry is amazing and is well worth the wait.

Chia Choc Granola

--

Chicken and Root Vegetable Broth
(Root Vegetable Broth with Tofu (V))

--

Chinese-style Chicken Stir-fry with Pak Choi
(Mushroom and Blackbean Stir-fry (V))

Day Three

Hooray for day 3! The lightest days are over and it gets easier from here. There are more carbohydrates in your evening meal and chocolate is officially allowed! It's worth jumping on the scales at the start of day 3. If you're on track I would expect you to have lost 2-4 pounds already.

Chia Choc Granola

--

Vegetable Chilli

--

Chicken Cassoulet
(Moroccan Spiced Eggs (V))

Day Four

By day 4 you should be getting into the spirit of the diet. You'll know what to expect and because you've made it this far you know you can make it to the end. Dinner is an absolute treat tonight!

Chia Choc Granola

--

Mexican Chicken Soup
(Mexican Bean Soup (V))

--

Lightly Spiced Prawns with Vegetable Rice
(Fresh Saag Paneer (V))

Day Five

Past the half way point and cruising to victory. How much weight have you lost so far?

Chia Choc Granola

--

Vegetable Chilli

--

Peanut Butter and Lime Prawns
(Feta Stuffed Red Peppers (V))

Day Six

Nearly at the finish line but don't get distracted by the weekend. It would be a tragedy to give up now. So stay strong and it's only one weekend.

Chia Choc Granola

--

Mexican Chicken Soup
(Mexican Bean Soup (V))

--

Chicken Cassoulet
(Moroccan Spiced Eggs (V))

Day Seven

Last day today. Don't lose your way now. Avoid Sunday dinners. Think of those weighing scales tomorrow morning. That is your goal.

Chia Choc Granola

--

Vegetable Chilli

--

Creamy Baked Salmon with New Potatoes and Mange Tout
(Bean Burgers with New Potatoes and Mange Tout (V))

BONUSES

As a special thank you for purchasing the '7 Day Detox' programme, I've got some amazing bonuses to get you started.

Bonus 1: 1-2-3 Get Ready to Detox Guide

Bonus 2: Take Me to the Shops

Bonus 3: Bonus Recipes - Feta and Avocado Salad + Mushroom Stuffed Peppers

All these bonuses are ready and waiting for you here:

www.52recipes.co.uk/7days/

Index

A

B

C

D

E

Printed in Great Britain
by Amazon